IMAGE
In The Mirror

Tommy Arnez

authorHOUSE®

AuthorHouse™
1663 Liberty Drive
Bloomington, IN 47403
www.authorhouse.com
Phone: 1-800-839-8640

Published by AuthorHouse   03/23/2012

ISBN: 978-1-4685-7321-3 (sc)
ISBN: 978-1-4685-7323-7 (hc)
ISBN: 978-1-4685-7322-0 (e)

Library of Congress Control Number: 2012905478

CONTENTS

All the information contained in this book comes from years of research and hard work. My goal has always been to be the best image maker I can possibly be. Many thanks to those who have afforded me the privilege of working with their hair and to those who believed in me. To the reader, thank you for giving me the opportunity to provide information so that when you see your image in the mirror, what you find is your own true uniqueness.

My prayer is that the readers will find this book helpful and enlightening, and as a result of appreciating the differences of God's creation, celebrate the beauty that lies within all of us.

DEDICATION

This book is dedicated to:

Desiree Hoard—my beloved wife and best friend. You have been my constant supporter. Thank you for your patience, understanding, and input in making this book become a reality. You are truly a gift from God! He knew exactly what I needed when He created you. My love for you grows stronger each day. You truly are the "glue" that keeps me together!

Alberta Gipson—my late grandmother, who always made me feel special, taught me the importance of hard work, and told me to always strive to be the best I could be, no matter what I pursued.

Doris Gipson—my late mother, who always believed in me and encouraged me to pursue my dream.

PREFACE

Few people really discover their passion in life, and I am grateful to have discovered mine. I find great value in what I do because I am an image maker!

As far back as I can remember, I dreamed of being a hair designer. I did not want to be just another hair stylist; because my greatest desire was to use my creative abilities to help others look and feel their best.

By the time I made it to college my focus had shifted, and I pursued a degree in marketing instead. Soon after stumbling upon an article written about the legendary Vidal Sassoon, however, something in me sparked, and my fire was relit. I wholeheartedly began following my original dream.

Like Vidal Sassoon, I decided to pursue hair design, and following my grandmother's advice, my goal was to be my absolute best. I sought and received the best training available at that time and studied hard to be at the top of my profession.

Today I'm not only an educator but also a salon owner of more than thirty years. I have had the honor of making people look their best and the privilege of training others in my field to do the same. From my early days as a designer, I had a passion to share with others the knowledge I acquired. When I became an educator, passion met reality.

I'm thankful for the many doors that have opened for me. I've been blessed to work with many renowned designers and for several reputable organizations, including an international hair care company.

My numerous experiences have allowed me to learn about and work with all hair types and many different nationalities.

The thoughts and ideas shared in this book have been tested and proven on thousands, and I'm honored to be able to share some of what I have learned with you. In an industry that is constantly evolving, there is always so much more to learn. What I am sharing here with you will only scratch the surface.

As an educator, my mind is always open to new ideas and better ways to serve my clients. This book is a culmination of years of hard work and dedication to my profession.

Acknowledgments

Tommy Sharell & Cedric Dale Hoard, my two sons—you have both given me so much joy as I have watched you grow from babies to boys and from boys to men. I believe that God has great things planned for both of you. I am so proud of you and love you greatly.

Lisa Hightire—thank you for inspiring me to get started on this book and for the numerous hours you sacrificed laboring as if it were your own. May God abundantly bless you and your family!

My valued clients—thank you for giving me the opportunity to serve you and for putting your trust in me.

INTRODUCTION

Over the years I have had hundreds and maybe even thousands of verbal consultations with individuals about their hair. This book is being written in question-and-answer format, as I desire to draw you, the reader, into the conversation. I want you to feel like you are part of the dialogue. Imagine yourself sitting with friends, having questions about your hair, but not knowing whom to ask or even how to ask them. This book is designed to answer some of those questions. Please join Lisa Hightire, a longtime client, and I as we examine this inexhaustible subject together.

As you read, my desire is that you develop a greater understanding and appreciation of your own individual hair type while celebrating your own unique *Image in the Mirror*.

Tommy Arnez

Chapter 1

HAIR: IT'S ALL ABOUT TEXTURE

L: Tommy, there are so many different words in our society to describe hair—fine, thin, kinky, thick, straight, curly, and so on. As a professional, when you think of hair, what words or images come to mind?

T: I think of hair as a fabric and place it in two categories: textures and types. When I refer to hair *texture*, that represents the way hair feels to the touch: fine, medium, or coarse. When I refer to hair *type*, I am referring to the way the hair looks: straight, wavy, curly, or excessively curly. These two categories exist within every race.

When I use the terms *fine, medium,* and *coarse,* keep in mind that this indicates the diameter (size) of the hair strand. To help you better understand, let's think about the following three types of fiber: thread, yarn, and rope. When we compare these to our three hair textures, the thread is the thinnest (fine) fiber. Yarn is the middle (medium) fiber, which has greater flexibility and bends more easily than thread. And finally, rope (coarse) doesn't have much flexibility at all and certainly won't bend as easily as yarn. With this in mind, you get a better picture of the various textures of hair.

L: Which hair is the most ideal?

T: All hair textures can be ideal. It's just a matter of understanding how to manage the particular hair texture you have. Many hair designers would consider the medium texture (yarn) as more ideal.

L: Why? I thought you would say that fine hair is more ideal.

T: Society has preconditioned you to think that way. As I stated earlier, medium hair texture is considered most ideal because, like yarn, it is the most flexible, and you can do more with it.

L: That makes so much sense. If hair is fine, it's usually limp, and coarse hair can be very stiff. I get it!

T: Yes. Using this analogy will bring greater understanding as to what each texture is capable of producing. Again, no one texture is better than the other. It's just a matter of knowing exactly what to do with each hair type in order to create something beautiful. For example, fine hair texture can be one of the most challenging to manage because the diameter of the hair strand would be considered too thin and limp. The medium texture, on the other hand, has more flexibility, whereas the coarse texture would be more rigid and stiff. Coarse hair feels wiry, is thick, and holds curl for days because it's hardened and has a lot of protein in it. Remember that all races have fine, medium, and coarse hair, but the structure of the hair itself may be different.

L: This is interesting. Could you elaborate on how you would work with these different hair types? For example, how would you create more body with fine hair?

T: Very good question. Hair has three layers, the cuticle (outer layer), cortex (middle layer), and the medulla (inner layer). Fine hair is limp because it has just two of the three layers. It has the cuticle and cortex, but the medulla is missing. Fine hair also has less protein, which provides strength for hair, but more moisture than other hair types. (More detail on hair layers in chapter 2.)

In order to create more body for individuals with fine hair, there are a number of different approaches. One option would be adding curl to the hair by perming. A perm will add texture, which aids in adding the needed body to fine, limp hair. A second option would be to use shampoos, conditioners, and styling products specifically designed to help create more body and plump up the volume of the hair. A third option is to employ specific cutting techniques that help create body and volume. This, of course, depends on what the hair type is: straight, wavy, or curly. Although curly and wavy hair can also be fine in diameter, they have more texture than straight hair, so the hair type must also be considered.

L: Now I'm beginning to understand. Tommy, would you agree that in corporate America and society as a whole, straight hair is perceived as more acceptable and mainstream?

T: Typically when we look at society, it is common to see straight hair, and this is true with all ethnicities. For whatever reason, people seem to prefer having straight hair. For example, many use implements such as flat irons and chemicals to straighten their hair. The millions of dollars spent on these products further prove this point.

I believe it's because the styles and trends of today are different than they were some years ago. From a professional perspective, and working with various hair textures on a daily basis, I have seen so many trends come and go over the years. Although straightening the hair is really nothing new, history has a way of repeating itself, and this is just a period of time where the styles are once again focused on the straighter look. However, this is an individual choice. Any style is acceptable as long as it makes you feel good about yourself.

The main reason people like to alter their hair type or texture is because it becomes more flexible and more styling options become available. When people with fine, limp hair perm it, they alter their hair, making it more manageable and giving it flexibility. Those with excessively curly hair will often straighten it, making it more manageable in their eyes. These are all options available and are based on individual preference.

The reason I use the word *option* is because it gives individuals a wide range of choices to create a certain look with their particular hair texture. For example, if individuals have curly or excessively curly hair, they may love their texture, yet having it straightened gives them another styling option. The same holds true for people with straight hair. Perming is an option they can use to create curl. It's all about options.

These choices allow people to change the style of their hair for greater versatility. Options allow you to create different effects that will change your appearance and become an integral part of your fashion statement.

Everyone, no matter what their ethnicity, desires to have what they perceive to be the ideal texture of hair. By understanding what options are available, we can take what we historically and culturally think of as the worst hair and alter it to make it manageable and more beautiful. We can also take what we think of as the best hair texture and do exactly the same thing! Both are being altered for greater versatility of style.

L: Tommy, that is so interesting. So you are saying that women from all cultures really have more in common than they realize. All of us strive for the exact same thing when it comes to our hair—beauty and manageability.

T: Lisa, being a professional hair designer and educator gives me the opportunity to travel and work with so many different hair types. From Middle Eastern and African American to Asian and European—I've had the privilege of working with them all!

L: All are different with unique characteristics and each is to be appreciated.

T: Correct. From my personal observation, each race has some form of heavy texture. When I use the term *heavy*, I'm referring to the curl pattern in the hair, not necessarily the weight of the hair. With each curl pattern comes a different feel. Some are smooth, some soft, while others may be coarser. Generally speaking, the curl pattern of European and Hispanic women is looser than that of Middle Eastern and African American.

African hair is very heavily textured. If you think about it, the sun's rays are strong in Africa, and the heavy curl pattern of the hair protects the scalp from those rays. God is awesome! He knew what He was doing when He created the different hair textures for protection as well as beauty.

L: African Americans are essentially African, but their hair seems different. How is that?

T: You have to think about the blending of the races. When different genes come together, new textures are created! For example, the hair textures among the African Americans range from very, very curly to completely straight.

Again, when God created this world, He knew exactly what He was doing. He made people of various colors from various regions, and He designed us with our own unique texture. So we have to learn to appreciate and accept the uniqueness of each texture. That's why it really bothers me when I hear someone say, "I have bad, kinky, or nappy hair." No one has bad hair. It's just different. It's how you work with your hair that makes it exciting and beautiful, and this includes leaving it in its natural state.

L: That word *nappy* seems to have a negative connotation.

T: I've read that the root of the word *nappy* originated in England and referred to the nap of an animal's undercoat, meaning its fur. American slave owners adopted the term and began using it to refer to their slaves' hair. It is indeed a derogatory term, and that is why I refuse to use it to describe the texture of my African American or Middle Eastern clients. I prefer the term *excessively curly* because it more accurately describes this type of hair. And their hair is certainly not like an animal's fur.

L: Does the same stand true for the term *kinky*?

T: Absolutely. The word *kinky* is an American term referring to a knot, and all textures can become knotted. So the word *kinky* should be removed from your vocabulary as well.

L: That is so insightful. These words are used all the time. I never realized just how derogatory they can be. Now, I'll start looking at hair from a different perspective. Let's reiterate what you have just said. Hair is hair, regardless of nationality, and should be embraced as something beautiful and appreciated.

T: Right. A person's hair can actually be viewed as an accessory.

L: Wow. I never thought of it that way.

T: Yes. This is because fashion dictates hairstyles. And your hair is an accessory to complement your personal style.

L: You're right! Accessories, fabric, and fashion all go together. I never linked them to hair. Could you elaborate more on fabric and how it relates to hair?

T: Certainly. To illustrate, let's look at wool, cotton, and silk. Each one of these fabrics has a unique texture and, therefore, each serves a particular purpose. Cotton can be worn in the summer and winter. Wool is a winter fabric and keeps you warm. That doesn't mean that wool is a bad fabric because it's a heavier, coarser fabric. It serves its purpose as well as silk.

Many times when we look at straight hair, we think of it as silky and shiny. It is perceived as *good hair*. However, its *goodness* is predicated on the health of the hair, not on how straight it is. Good hair is healthy hair! Damaged hair, on the other hand, lacks shine because the outer layer has been negatively affected. When the outer layer isn't healthy, it gives hair a frizz, making it dull and lifeless.

Just as you should use different care instructions when working with different fabrics, you should use appropriate styling products, tools, and techniques for different hair textures. Just as fabric plays a vital role in fashion with regard to the different seasons, different hair textures play a role as an accessory in a person's fashion statement. One hair texture is neither superior nor inferior to another just as one fabric is not better or worse than another.

L: This is good. I have not thought about hair in this way before. Your explanation really simplifies the age-old *good hair/bad hair* myth.

T: There is a whole spectrum of differences in a society when it comes to hair. Asian hair is one of the strongest of all races. It's very straight, but even though it's straight, it can be very coarse. The texture can be very challenging if one isn't knowledgeable in how to work with it. Just because it's straight doesn't necessarily mean it's manageable and easy to work with.

L: Wow! That's so interesting. All I see is their super-straight hair, but have never considered its texture.

T: The cuticle is so thick and compact that the hair just hangs straight. How do you take something so straight, coarse, and compact, and make it bend? You alter the texture. Texture can be altered by using different types of cutting techniques that make it more manageable, fluid, and flowing. And here again, you've created more options with that particular texture. Asian hair can also be relaxed to help manage its coarseness.

L: It doesn't look coarse at all. Does it feel coarse?

T: No. If it does feel coarse or rough, it could be that the cuticle layer has been damaged, giving it a rough feel. But that can happen to anyone's hair. When we think of coarse, we should think of its thickness versus how it feels. Some African American hair is coarse and thick based on genetics, but basically, the average African American's hair is not always strong. Asian hair is very strong and can withstand more. The color of Asian hair is typically black, which makes it more difficult to color.

L: Is African American hair weak in its natural state?

T: Yes. And when chemical is applied, the hair becomes even weaker. When a relaxer is used, the result is the actual shrinking and thinning of the cuticle of the hair. That's why it's so important that hair be conditioned with protein and moisture to strengthen it. It is critical to shampoo at least once weekly to restore what has been removed. But one should always be mindful of the individual needs of his or her own hair and shampoo and cleanse it accordingly.

L: So, theoretically, the more we shampoo, the more we restore what chemical processes strip out?

T: You've got it! If a person gets a relaxer every six to eight weeks, it's robbing his or her hair of protein, moisture, and fatty acids. If people only shampoo every two weeks, they are not restoring enough of these essential elements prior to their next treatment. They are only putting back what's essential to make the hair healthy three times. But if people wash their hair at least once every week, they replace the necessary elements six times. When you shampoo and condition your hair, you're putting back what's been stripped away by the chemical process. It's very, very important to maintain the healthiness of the hair. You must put back what the chemical processing takes away. I can never stress that enough. We don't want hair to become damaged or dull so the hair constantly requires restoration.

What I want you to take away from this chapter is the importance of understanding that hair is hair. One hair type is not superior to another. One texture is not better than another. There are many options available for every texture. It's all up to you!!!

Chapter 2

THE COMPOSITION FACTOR

We previously discussed texture and developed a better understanding and appreciation of all hair types. It is equally important that we understand the composition of hair so we know how to treat it and maintain it.

Hair is composed of oil, protein, and water. Oil is the essential fatty acid that naturally lubricates. Protein, also known as keratin, acts as the hair strengthener, while water provides hydration. What makes the hair strand healthy is a balance of both protein and moisture. Hair consists of three layers: the cuticle, the cortex, and the medulla. The cuticle is the outer layer that serves as protection for the cortex. The cortex is the inner layer where protein and moisture are found. The medulla, usually missing in fine hair, is the third, innermost layer.

When protein is missing, the hair becomes weak. When we look at hair, it's important to note that thicker and coarser hair has more protein in it. Medium hair has a balance of both protein and moisture. Fine hair has moisture but lacks protein, which means, and this is regardless of race, it has something crucial missing for its manageability.

If the hair lacks protein, it is often fine, weak, and limp because, again, protein strengthens hair. In essence, it hardens the hair. I don't want to give the impression that this concept of *hardening* is negative. When you have weak, brittle fingernails, they lack protein and need something to strengthen them. It works the same way with hair. We want fine hair to be strong, because the stronger it is, the better it will hold its style. Protein must be added to the hair in order to make it balanced. The hair already has moisture, so adding a strengthener will balance it out.

Medium-textured hair is considered the ideal texture because it's balanced, and when healthy it contains both protein and moisture, which makes it beautiful and flexible. When we see hair that has movement and body, it's simply because it has flexibility. It has a balance of protein and moisture. Although ideal, if not properly cared for, this particular hair texture can become damaged, primarily through the use of chemicals. For example, relaxers, permanent waves, or colors rob the hair of vital nutrients—moisture and protein. The composition of the hair changes because chemicals deplete moisture and protein in the hair. These nutrients must be restored.

Allow me to get technical for a moment as I believe that individuals utilizing chemical services needs to understand what is actually happening to their hair. A relaxer is highly caustic (corrosive), and it dries and weakens the hair. The pH of the relaxer is highly alkaline. When hair becomes highly alkaline, it has to be offset by restoring it back to its proper pH (4.5-5.5 on the pH scale).

L: What exactly is the pH scale?

T: Simply stated, pH stands for potential Hydrogen. It's a scale ranging from zero to fourteen used by manufacturers to determine the acidic and alkalinity levels in a particular hair product. This is why it's important to have a professional work with your hair. When you use products that have high pH levels, it puts the health of one's hair at risk.

On the pH scale, one to six is considered acidic. Products with low acidic levels keep the hair shiny and healthy by keeping the cuticle layer of the hair closed, retaining the protein and moisture. Seven is neutral. Anything above seven is alkaline. Alkaline opens the cuticle layer, exposing the cortex, and causing the depletion of protein and moisture. Products that are highly alkaline rob the hair of its healthiness. Healthy hair should be somewhere within the 4.5 to 5.5 range on the pH scale.

L: How can a person know what the pH of his or her hair is?

T: You can't really test or see hair pH, but you can tell whether it's in the healthy range by how it feels and whether or not it reflects natural shine.

Because a relaxer is a chemical itself, it goes into the hair and restructures it, changing the integrity of the hair and causing the hair to become weak. If not properly applied or if left on longer than the manufacturer's recommendations, the relaxer itself has been known to literally eat the hair away, resulting in severe breakage.

L: Yikes! Tommy, I shudder to think of all the home-relaxers and other treatments people apply themselves!

T: I know. Chemical processes should always be applied by an experienced, licensed professional because we are dealing with a precarious substance. Let me give you an example to better illustrate what a relaxer can do. Denim is very strong. If you give a pair of new jeans to a boy who constantly crawls on the floor, what happens to the knee over a period of time?

L: The fabric begins to wear and tear.

T: Exactly. That's what happens to hair too. When chemicals are improperly applied or left on too long, over a period of time, the fibers of the hair weaken and eventually breakage occurs.

Additionally, anytime you apply a chemical to the hair, it has the potential of coming in contact with the skin and causing chemical burns.

If the chemical can damage the skin, imagine what it can do to the hair. If a chemical is left on too long, it is going to cause the hair to feel mushy and go into the stage referred to as *redox*. Redox means the hair has gone beyond stretching ability. This means the hair is *completely destroyed.*

L: Wow. That is very sobering. Are there other chemicals that can damage the hair?

T: Yes. Let's touch on permanent waving. I mentioned earlier that this is another option to alter the texture of the hair. But just like relaxing, it can be damaging as well. There are primarily two types of perms—an alkaline or acid wave. Alkaline perms are used without heat and the pH is typically higher. Damage can occur if the hair is not wrapped properly with a perm rod. If the perm rod is wrapped too tight, it places stress on the hair and the solution can cause breakage. You can also over process it by leaving it on too long.

An acid wave is used with heat. A test curl must be done in both cases. Again, if the hair is not properly wrapped with perm rods, breakage will occur. Because the perm solution is a liquid, if the skin around the hairline and neck is not properly protected, severe burns may occur. So again, these types of services should always be performed by a professional.

Lightening the hair, commonly referred to as bleaching, can also do severe damage. Understanding the process of lightening is important. Every person has primary colors in his or her hair, and they are blue, red, and yellow. When lightening hair, the first of the primary colors to leave is blue. Red is second. And if the hair is taken to the platinum stage (the whitest blonde), the last of the primaries to leave is yellow. In these cases the natural pigment or melanin is being dispersed.

Let me explain what I mean by this. If you were to break a thermometer, the mercury would disperse into particles, meaning it would completely separate. Picturing this analogy, the hair pigment can be completely dispersed if the lightening process is left on too long. The integrity of the hair is jeopardized because of the many stages it has been subjected to, and the hair has been robbed of its protein and moisture.

This is especially true if the hair has already been chemically treated or it's not strong enough to receive this type of treatment. Again, all lightening services should be performed with caution and by a licensed professional who has a thorough understanding of the type of hair that is receiving these services.

Coloring the hair, although different than lightening, is still a chemical process. The chemical penetrates, changing the molecular structure of the hair. You are lifting and depositing a different color, changing the natural tone or level. By level I'm referring to shade, which ranges from the darkest (1) to the lightest (10).

To illustrate, if a person's hair is light brown, which is a level five, and you're trying to achieve light blonde, which is a level eight, the peroxide needed to lighten and deposit the desired shade needs to be at a high volume. So you have to alter the pigment in the hair to create a new color. The important thing with all services is how the hair is treated and what is used with the hair after any service is performed. In all cases, the hair needs to be rebuilt, and protein and moisture need to be replenished in order to keep the hair healthy. That is why it's so critical that services of this magnitude always be performed by a licensed professional who is knowledgeable not only about hair type and texture, but chemicals as well.

When a chemical service is applied to a client's hair based on manufacturer directions, as a professional, we know we've removed some of the protein and moisture, opening the cuticle layer of the hair and changing the hair's pH level. So while the cuticle layer is open, we have to immediately restore the hair back to a healthy state.

Because alkalinity leaves the cuticle open, we now have to infuse the hair with a low pH shampoo and conditioner in order to restore protein and moisture and bring it back to the acidic stage. The protein and moisture must be broken down into molecular size in order to absorb into the hair and repair it. This is why you cannot use just any random product on the hair. The licensed professional should instruct the client on a home maintenance regiment in order to maintain the health of the hair between salon visits.

L: From a retail standpoint, why does the term *pH balanced* no longer appear on shampoo labels?

T: Good question. The majority of professional products have maintained the pH label on the bottle. However, to answer your question, I believe that most of today's shampoos and conditioners are manufactured with a low pH level so they may no longer need to label the product as such. This may be an industry standard. Again, this is why it is absolutely crucial for clients to consult with their stylist.

Speaking from a professional perspective, pH balance can be misleading because the pH means the potential Hydrogen a shampoo offers. What you're looking for in a shampoo and conditioner is the acidic range. On the pH scale, the percentage of acidity is important. If too acidic, it shrinks the cuticle layer. A pH of 1 or 2 is very acidic and drying. A pH of 4.5-5.5 is the best acidic level, and this pH is healthiest for the hair. A pH 3 is excellent when the hair is high in alkaline. Hair itself doesn't have a pH level.

We determine the best pH range for individual's hair based on their oil and sweat glands. Oil and sweat glands are 4.5-5.5 in pH. The oil glands help lubricate the hair and protect it. Alkaline is drying to the hair. When shampoos were formulated years ago, they were highly alkaline, and alkalinity dried the hair out.

L: So, as you said, it's become an industry standard to make shampoos pH balanced in general?

T: Right. So when we are repairing hair, we need to use products that are going to help give the proper balance, which is 4.5-5.5. Again, whenever we're dealing with chemicals such as relaxers, permanent waves, and color, we need to replenish what has been depleted.

Additionally, the essential fatty acids in hair are removed, so we need to replace essential fatty acids in order for the composition of hair to be healthy. When we see someone with chemically treated hair and it looks shiny and healthy, we can believe that his or her hair has been properly maintained and the structure and integrity has been brought back to its healthy stage by the use of proper products on the hair. That's why it is so important to understand the shampoos and conditioners you use. Everything you choose for your hair should help maintain its health.

People experiment with chemical services at home without being fully aware of the consequences. In most cases they lack the knowledge and skill to properly perform such services.

Let me give you an example. If a person were to apply a chemical relaxer and not thoroughly rinse and properly neutralize the hair with a neutralizing shampoo, when the hair comes in contact with heat, the heat will reactivate the relaxer. Once the chemicals in the relaxer are reactivated, guess what's going to happen? That hair will *snap*! As with any fabric, whether silk, wool or cotton, you have to properly care for it. Your hair has to be properly cared for as well.

Since we're talking about the composition of hair, let's talk about the division of hair.

L: The division of hair? What's that?

T: When I say division of hair, I'm referring to the areas above and beneath the scalp. Above the scalp is the hair shaft and below the scalp we find the hair follicle. The hair shaft is connected to the hair follicle, and below the scalp, the follicle is connected to the hair root.

L: So you're saying that the root of the hair is actually below the scalp?

T: Yes. Most people say, "I need my roots touched up." What they are saying is really incorrect. The root is inside the scalp in the hair follicle. You cannot see the root. What's being retouched is the new growth, not the hair root. That's important for people to know.

If the hair follicle is pulled out of the scalp, it may never grow back. This often happens with weaving and people who wear their hair braided extremely tight. Remember, if the hair follicle is damaged, the hair may never grow back. In fact, the hair follicle is also a breeding ground for germs. That's why it is so important for the hair to be shampooed regularly. The purpose of shampooing is mainly to cleanse the scalp because a healthy scalp produces healthy hair.

L: Wow! Pairing a *healthy scalp* with *clean scalp* really makes me think about people who don't regularly wash their hair.

T: Yes, and you can also get what I call *scalp acne*, which is a condition that occurs when the pores of the scalp become clogged from sweat, dirt, and bacteria. As a professional, I see this often.

L: I've never thought that much about the health of my scalp. So when we sweat, it affects the scalp. And is it safe to assume that the odor that sometimes comes from the hair is connected to the pores of the scalp being clogged?

T: Absolutely. That is why it's important to shampoo regularly. Depending on your lifestyle and activities, some individuals may need to shampoo more often than others.

Getting back to the point of the pores of the scalp being clogged, your pores open up when they come in contact with chemical substances applied to the hair. This again is why proper application, removal, and shampooing of the chemical are essential. The goal is to thoroughly remove any residue that may have gotten trapped under the scalp of the hair.

L: How often should people shampoo their hair?

T: Well, the answer is simple really. How often do you *need* to shampoo it? If you're very active or work in an environment with smoke, food, or other fumes, you're going to want fresh-smelling, clean hair. Your hair is like a sponge and absorbs odors. If you're very active, you may have to shampoo daily.

L: Culturally, some wash their hair every day while others wash it only once or twice weekly. Speak to that.

T: It's a myth that every culture can't shampoo their hair every day. It's not shampooing that destroys the hair. Shampooing daily can actually be very good for the hair, no matter what culture an individual may come from. Shampooing is safe and gentle for the hair with the proper pH balance, and a conditioner can be very healthy for the hair, as long as it is free of harsh detergents and selected for your particular hair type.

Damage to the hair often occurs *after* it has been shampooed. The constant blow drying, curling, excessive heat, and combing practices are just a few of the things creating some of the many challenges to the hair.

L: How do you get around this?

T: Simply by changing methods. If you use a blow dryer and curling iron on hair every day, you're going to destroy the hair. Using a blow dryer on the highest setting places stress on hair, and this is especially true for chemically-treated hair. There are various techniques we can use to eliminate the stress. If you must use heat, instead of blow drying, consider roller setting, wrapping, sculpting, molding, and sitting under a hooded dryer. By doing this you are lessening the amount of damage and stress on the hair, thereby maintaining its healthiness. Of course, you could also let it air dry, if you prefer.

L: What's the difference in blow drying and sitting under the dryer? Heat is heat.

T: That's a good question. When we sculpt (molding hair in a desired direction), wrap (wrapping hair around the head while wet to create body), or put rollers in the hair, the hair is in a resting stage. Without the blow dryer, there's no stress caused by a comb or brush continually pulling on and placing tension on the hair. With a blow dryer, the heat is more concentrated, giving more opportunity for breakage and damage. Don't get me wrong. Blow drying in and of itself isn't bad, but proper usage is a major key to great results.

Sitting under the dryer is less stressful. We are eliminating wear and tear on the hair. Remember our denim analogy? With continual friction, eventually you will weaken the fabric. It is the same with your hair.

L: Interesting. I have another question about blow drying. How much is too much?

T: Over time, constant blow drying, the use of hot air, the comb, brush, flat iron, and curling can to lead to damage, so we need to eliminate the amount of stress placed on the hair in order to help maintain healthy hair.

L: Let's talk about stress and things in our lives that may impact the health of our hair.

T: Stress greatly impacts one's entire life, and it's important for us to learn to manage the many stresses of life. For example, you leave for a meeting that's fifty miles away and only give yourself ten minutes to get there. You are placing unnecessary stress upon yourself. When we are under stress, it affects our hair follicle, which ultimately affects the hair. There is a muscle, the *arrector pili*, that is connected to the hair follicle. When triggered by stress, this muscle, which is connected to your nerve, causes hair to appear to *stand up*. If stress continually triggers this muscle, it will often cause abnormal shedding of the hair.

The same holds true when stress comes as a result of illness. If the immune system breaks down or one is required to take certain medications, this muscle can affect the hair follicle, weakening it. When the hair follicle is negatively affected, often times the hair sheds or becomes lifeless because what affects the body internally affects the body externally.

For example, moisture continually evaporates from the body as well as the hair, so not only do we have to put moisture back into the hair with products, we must also drink plenty of water.

L: I don't believe I have ever related moisture in my hair to the amount of water I drink. I thought it came from oil I either applied or secreted.

T: Well, primarily, the body needs water. But when we talk about natural oil, there are a number of things that come into play. Our diet and what we put into our bodies, blood circulation, emotional disturbances, stimulation of our glands, and drugs all affect the natural oil production and secretion.

If we're taking medication, it can affect the natural oil production. Certain medication may deplete the right amounts of amino acids. Amino acids are the chemical units that make up protein. They are often known as protein's *building blocks*, and they affect the skin and hair, so it's important that we maintain proper balances. A healthy diet that includes fruits and vegetables, and getting the proper amounts of amino acids, helps produce natural oils in our scalp, keeping it healthy. It's the oils that actually help protect and condition our hair and scalp, but we must eat healthy foods.

L: I'm with you on that. Pizza has plenty of greasy cheese. And don't forget the burgers and fries!

T: Yeah, that diet is going to produce fat all right! I'm talking about eating healthy food on a regular basis. A healthy diet is not only going to keep a woman looking good and feeling great, but will also promote the growth of a healthy head of hair.

Blood circulation is another element to consider. If your blood is not circulating properly, it will affect the growth of your hair and its healthiness because blood nourishes the hair.

L: Seriously? Blood?

T: It is true. Someone once did a test where a person was injected with amino acid to see how long it would take for the acid to come out in the hair shaft. After one week the amino acid was detected at the base of the scalp and in the hair, so what we consume gets into the blood stream, flows throughout the body, and feeds the hair follicle and hair shaft.

It's important to note that what you consume can greatly affect the condition of your hair. So healthy blood flow, a well-balanced diet, drinking plenty of water, avoiding excessive stress, and getting adequate amounts of sleep and exercise all contribute to a healthy head of hair.

L: Hold it. Exercise!!?

T: That's right. Exercise helps to alleviate stress as well as maintain healthy blood circulation. A well-balanced diet and exercise regimen promote healthy hair. People wonder why they're having problems with their hair. The answer could lie in how well they take care of themselves. Many don't realize the correlation between health and wellness and healthy hair.

A lack of exercise or sleep deprivation will take its toll on the hair. Sleep plays an important role in allowing the body to repair and renew itself, and hair growth can be influenced by a lack of sleep. Changes in sleeping patterns have been shown to impact the body's immune function and physical and mental stamina. The hair is very sensitive to changes within the body, and hair loss is often the result of an internal disturbance.

To elaborate more on medication and/or drugs, there are various types prescribed by doctors, and it's important to know the side effects. Certain medicines can cause thinning of the hair and affect nutrients in the blood. Medications, such as those for thyroid problems or hypertension, can cause thinning of the hair, so check with your doctor or nutritionist to replenish the nutrients that medications may be depleting from your body.

L: How do we know what to eat or the proper supplements to take and in what amounts?

T: Consult with a nutritionist or your physician. No matter what form of medications you may be taking, always be aware of any changes in your hair. Diet, exercise, and medication all, in one way or another, affect one's emotional state, which also affects the hair.

L: The condition of our hair can be related to our emotional state?

T: Yes. It's natural for the body to respond to emotional stresses—however, prolonged stress could potentially cause problems for your hair. There are nerve endings in the scalp connected to the hair, which can affect the frontal hairline as well as the crown of the head, and this can often be attributed to hair loss in these areas. So remember, if it causes problems for the body, it could cause problems for your hair.

As you can see, there are a number of factors that can affect the body so you must be aware of the possible changes that may occur in your hair. This will help you better determine cause and effect and, upon consulting a professional hair stylist, develop a plan of treatment.

Chapter 3

WHAT IS HEALTHY AND WHAT ISN'T

In chapter 1, we covered the beauty in each texture. In chapter 2, we discussed the composition of the hair. Next, we will cover the various shapes of hair—straight, wavy, curly, and excessively curly—and how each grows from the scalp.

Typically, straight hair grows straight out of the scalp and curves, creating a rounded shape. Wavy hair grows with a slightly oval bend and has a bit more of a curve. Curly and excessively curly hair both grow in a spiral pattern, but excessively curly hair has a tighter pattern and lies flat and closest to the scalp.

L: This is good information. Tommy, I want to address the issue of oil in the hair. Many complain about their hair being too oily while others complain about it being too dry. Can you speak to this?

T: Certainly! The hair strand grows out of the hair follicle located below the scalp where the sebum (natural oil) is found. Regardless of ethnicity, straight hair grows straight out of the scalp. Straight hair produces more oil because the oil is able to move right through the scalp up to the hair strand. So an individual with straighter hair may have an oilier feel to the hair.

Like straight hair, the oils in wavy hair travel through the scalp, but because of the waves, the natural oils can't lubricate the hair as generously as straight hair. So individuals with wavy hair may have a normal oil balance to the hair.

Because curly and excessively curly hair grows out of the scalp in a tight spiral formation (laying flat on the scalp), natural oils have a more challenging time traveling up the hair shaft to lubricate it. For this reason, curly hair has a tendency to be dry, and excessively curly hair can be even drier, making it more challenging.

L: Challenging in terms of what?

T: It is a challenge to get moisture to the hair because of the way it grows. The tighter the curl, the more fragile the strand, and that's why excessively curly hair is more fragile than curly hair. It has weak points throughout the strand where curly hair does not.

L: Tommy, in your opinion, which hair is better? Would it be straight, wavy, curly, or excessively curly hair?

T: Because some believe that certain types of texture are considered good and others are considered bad, you've probably heard people say things like, "She or he has good hair" or "She or he has bad hair."

What they are referring to is the texture of an individual's hair. No one texture of hair is better than the other. Good hair is healthy hair. Bad hair is damaged hair.

L: Say that again!

T: Good hair is healthy hair. Bad hair is damaged hair. It's that simple. Regardless of whether the hair is straight, wavy, curly, or excessively curly, the health of the hair is not determined by texture, but by the condition of the hair.

L: Wow! This is liberating. Can you tell me what would appear to be the pros and cons of each hair texture?

T: Of course I can. All hair comes in various diameters, which is the size of the hair strand. And thick or fine, the hair strand can vary and will determine what the hair can or will do. Know this, regardless of race, if a person has straight hair, it can be fine, medium, or thick in diameter. I've personally encountered individuals of various races—Asian, Hispanic, Caucasian, African American, and Middle Eastern—who have fine, straight hair.

L: Do some find straight and fine hair to be problematic?

T: Many do, but it's actually easy to comb. Straight, fine hair may be challenging to style, and many with this hair type desire thicker hair with more body. Often times in order for them to be satisfied, they may need to seek the advice of a professional. They may consider having their texture altered with perming services and/or certain cutting techniques to help enhance their texture.

L: That's interesting. You've covered fine, straight hair. Now, let's talk about straight hair that's medium in diameter.

T: The person with this hair type has a bit more flexibility because it has more bend and manageability and holds a better curl. Because of the flexibility in its bend, it yields a little more control in its style. Medium, straight hair has to have the right cut because the haircut will help create volume and lift. This individual wouldn't necessarily need a perm because a proper cut will give this hair the manageability it needs without chemicals. Without the right haircut and styling tools, this individual will become frustrated, much like the person with straight, fine hair. It's a matter of knowing exactly what to do with the hair and seeking professional advice from someone who thoroughly understands hair texture.

L: Straight, thick hair?

T: For most individuals the most challenging hair type is straight and thick because it's coarse in texture. It is said to be more challenging because it's stiff and has little-to-no flexibility. Ordinarily, people with this hair type have difficulty managing it on their own because it just hangs. Once again, the right haircut will alter the texture and create the desired mobility. Typically, the type of instrument used to create that texture and mobility is a razor, and it requires skill in order to achieve the desired texture. Again, this is why it's important to consult with a professional.

So for all of those who believed that straight hair is *good* hair, you now know that *good* hair has more to do with health than it does with texture.

L: This is such good information, and I've learned so much. Let's talk about wavy and curly hair.

T: Believe it or not, there are different degrees of waviness: tight, medium, and loose. I'm not going to discuss so much the diameter, but I am going to focus on the three types of waves. A person with wavy hair automatically has body because of the texture of the hair. So let's discuss the person who has tight, wavy hair. The person with this hair type is often dissatisfied because it is hard to keep straight. It's prone to frizzing. Even when straightened with an implement, it won't stay straight. No matter what you do, you can never completely remove the wave. In this case, relaxing the hair or using a straightening agent will give the hair more control over the frizz because they loosen the wave pattern. Ultimately, if you have the right products, this hair type can be fun to style in its natural state with beautiful results.

Hair with a medium wave pattern looks great in its natural state. The disadvantage is if you try to straighten it with a flat iron or blow dry and curl, the style doesn't last as long because the wave pattern is so strong. Just like the person with the tighter wave pattern, you may want to consider relaxing the hair.

I want you to understand that one does not have to be a certain race to have a certain hair type. The characteristics I've mentioned are common to all nationalities. It's important to grasp this concept in terms of texture, *not* ethnicity. My hope is that this information destroys the myth that certain hair textures are associated with certain races. Regardless of which hair type you have, you will appreciate the uniqueness that is you. As a professional, I've seen all textures in nearly every race.

The very loose wavy hair type has more style options than the other two, and also looks great in its natural state. You can set it with rollers, blow dry, flat iron, or use a curling iron to give the hair a smoother look. The person with this hair type has more flexibility because the hair is a lot easier to change or style, which gives the person more options.

L: It seems like straightening the hair is the goal here for the best texture!

T: Not necessarily. It's a matter of one's personal preference. I want to convey that just because a person's hair is straight, wavy, or curly doesn't make it ideal, because every hair type has its advantages and disadvantages.

Educating ourselves is important so we can explore various options choosing the best solutions for our own individual hair type.

L: Tommy, let's talk about curly hair.

T: Certainly. There are different degrees of curl, just as there are different degrees of waviness. Let's focus on curly and excessively curly hair. We will begin with curly hair. When we think of curly hair, we envision soft, loose curls. This is the type of hair that people will generally look at and say, "That's good hair." What they're really looking at is the texture. Curly hair doesn't require a lot of management, and when allowed to air dry with its natural curl, it will stand out. You can run your fingers through it, and with the right haircut, it will be even more pronounced. Just because a person's hair is curly, doesn't mean it's good. If it's not in great condition, it could potentially be damaged. Don't be deceived by appearance.

If curly hair is not properly cared for, it has a tendency to be dry, but it also has advantages that other hair types do not. For instance, the curl itself looks great if it's shiny and healthy. You don't have to change the hair, making it straight—you can simply wear it curly, in its natural state.

The next curl texture I want to cover is excessively curly. Excessively curly is commonly referred to in negative or demeaning terms like *kinky* or *nappy*. It can be demeaning to some because of what these terms imply. *Kinky* is defined as something tight or twisted, while *nappy* is a derogatory term made famous in the late 1800s and early 1900s when referring to the hair of people of African descent. The hair is not kinky or nappy; it is actually excessively curly. We have to be mindful of how our words impact people's self-image. When we use negative words to define ourselves, it negatively affects the way we view ourselves. It's important for people with excessively curly hair to understand that their hair is extremely curly, not nappy or kinky.

Historically, there were individuals of a certain ethnicity brought to the US who were stripped of their culture and customs. There were no combs or brushes designed for their hair type, and therefore they tried to assimilate. There was very little knowledge or understanding at that time of how to properly care for this hair type.

This is one of the most misunderstood types of hair and probably the most abused by those within the culture itself. Many individuals are unhappy with it and greatly desire to change because society has made them feel that their hair is inferior. They don't fit in, and their hair type doesn't belong in what would be considered the mainstream. I find many are resorting to hair extensions or implementing weaves of other hair types, trying to fit in to achieve what is considered to be the ideal hair. It's all in an effort to feel good about themselves. I'm not saying this is bad, but I am saying we have to learn to work with and appreciate what we have.

You can look and feel your best by simply educating yourself and properly caring for your own God-given head of hair. Your sense of worth can't be based on who you are not or what you don't have. It has to be based on who you are and what you have been given by God. Take what you have and make it the best it can be. Don't worry if your hair doesn't grow long or it's not the texture you desire. Learn to embrace and enhance what you have! With today's modern technology, there are so many advances in tools and techniques that can be used to style this type of hair.

In my profession, I've seen a number of ethnic groups with curly hair. It's not just limited to one race. It would surprise you to see the number of women who struggle with the notion that their hair is nappy or kinky. Instead of viewing it as excessively curly, it's viewed as problematic. Because I'm a professional and I enjoy working with all hair types, I embrace the challenge to educate individuals on the importance of loving their hair, no matter what type or texture they may have.

I've seen excessively curly hair among the Italians, Middle Eastern, people of African descent, as well as Europeans. Typically, people only notice it in those of African descent, and this hair type is not bad. It can be very good if it is healthy. It is important for hair care professionals to clearly understand all hair types and textures to enhance its beauty and styling options. God created all hair, and nothing He created is bad. All hair textures are beautiful because they reflect God's creativity.

There are many advantages to having excessively curly hair. If you decide to chemically straighten it, it has a tremendous amount of body, and this type of hair has a natural crimp that affords numerous styling options. Excessively curly hair can be very fun to work with. In its natural state it can be straightened, braided, styled into dreadlocks, or twisted. These are all options someone with excessively curly hair can explore.

Hopefully you are able to see that healthy hair is based on the condition of the hair and not what we have historically thought it to be. My desire is to help you see hair from a different perspective. Regardless of its texture, one is not better than another. They are just different!

Chapter 4

IMAGE IS EVERYTHING

As previously stated, I view myself as an *image maker,* and as such, I've come to recognize the importance that individuals' image plays in how others view them, and more importantly, how they view themselves.

Hollywood plays a vital role in influencing the images that we typically see and desire to achieve. It presents all styles of hair. From actresses and singers to performers, the majority of what is presented is usually long and flowing. Occasionally you'll see individuals who go against the grain and choose to wear their hair shorter, or you may see someone with curly hair or dreadlocks, but for the most part, what you see coming out of Hollywood is long, full, and flowing.

A person does not necessarily have to buy extensions to make it longer, but in our society millions of dollars are spent in an effort to lengthen the hair when individuals can simply learn to care for and maximize their own.

Consider creating your own image based on your individuality or uniqueness. Let's focus on creating an image for the unique person that you are.

What is your skin color? What is your hair like? What color are your eyes? Do you know your body shape? Did you know that your hair, eyes, and skin tone each play an important part in creating the image that is uniquely you?

Let me give you an example. The proportion of your body and hairstyle should be aesthetically balanced for your body type. Your hairstyle should fit your body type.

L: When you say *body type*, what do you mean?

T: Your shape, whether it's pear, round, etc.

L: That's what I thought you meant, but honestly, I didn't think you'd consider body types because you're not necessarily in the fashion world.

T: Yes. I've been trained to take into consideration the person's total image. Posture should also be considered when creating a hairstyle. If an individual slumps when standing, he or she should not wear a cut that's slanted forward because it drags them down, causing them to appear even more slumped.

L: Wow! So how do you assess this when you have a client?

T: When a client first walks in, I've trained myself to subtly observe their posture. Although I may encourage a client to allow me to style their hair one way, they may be adamant about having it another way. It may not be the best styling option for them, so I have to compromise by honoring their request while at the same time merging what I know will look best for them.

Let's say a tall, thin woman with a very long neck comes into the salon and requests a short haircut such as a bob. If the bob she requests is round in shape, she will look like a lollypop. Now, this may sound humorous, but it's important for you to visualize my point.

As an image maker, I must always consider the coordination of an individual's physical body, face structure, and posture (aesthetic balance or proportion) in order to bring out the best in that individual.

Let's look at another example. If a female has a wide neck and broad shoulders and she requests to have her hair cut short with the back shaped as a square, it's going to expose the neck, giving it a wider appearance. The end result will have her looking like a football player, and that's not what we want. A lady should always look soft and feminine.

L: For this particular body shape, what would enhance her femininity?

T: The best line to create a softer look for this body type is an oval or 'v' shape in the back. This will diminish the appearance of a wide neck.

Here's an illustration that I would like for you, the reader, to participate in. I often use this illustration with my peers or colleagues when training on the topic of balance and proportion.

If you look at a one dollar bill, you will find a picture of President George Washington on the front of it. Looking at his face and hair you can clearly see that the hairstyle doesn't complement his facial features. The balance of the hairstyle is not in proportion to his personal features. It actually accentuates the size of his nose and the wideness of his forehead, and gives his face a longer look. President Washington needed a hairstyle that would complement his appearance instead of enhancing what would be considered to be facial flaws. This is not to disrespect President Washington in any way. It's just an illustration I use to get you to see how important it is to make sure the hairstyle and cut complement the client.

Now I want to talk about the profile or the side view of the face. The profile of a person actually helps you create a hairstyle. We typically see a person's profile more than we see the front of the face. When you're sitting next to someone, you don't see the front of his or her face; you see his or her profile. If someone is walking with you side by side, he or she sees the overall profile of your face and body. This is important because your profile actually determines your overall facial and body proportion.

Allow me go into greater detail. If you pull your hair away from your face, you can get a clearer perspective. What you want to do is start by looking from the hairline to the eye, from the eye to the nose, and from the nose to the chin. This helps you determine which areas are wider or longer, and by understanding this, you can see what needs to be balanced.

If you are wider from the hairline to the eye, your hairline sits farther back, and you will want a style to balance a protruding forehead. In other words, your facial features should appear in balance from your hairline to your eyes, from your eyes to your nose tip, and from your nose tip to your chin.

Now, let's look at the front of the face. Because we're not perfect, did you know our features are also imperfect? For example, one of our eyes is higher than the other. Even our nose and ears are not balanced. As an image maker, this knowledge is vital when designing a hairstyle. It also helps determine which side to part the hair on based on how low or high the eye is. The hair part should be placed on the side where the eye is lowest, because a part gives the illusion of the eye being raised and thus brings it into balance. If the hair is hanging next to the eye that's lower, it's going to make the eye look even lower.

There are also individuals with very close-set eyes or with wide-set eyes. Wide-set eyes are far apart from the bridge of the nose. With close-set eyes, when the hairstyle frames the face, it pushes the eyes even closer together, giving them the *bead-eyed* look. On the other hand, the person with wide-set eyes shouldn't have the hair pulled away from the face because it makes the eyes appear even farther apart.

L: Tommy, you mean to tell me that you're able to take all this in when a client walks through the door and sits in your chair?

T: Yes. Again, I'm trained and have trained others to decipher the fine details of balance in image making.

L: That's good information. Can we talk about the profile of the body and its role in all of this?

T: Certainly. The reason I mentioned the profile of your body is because it enables you to see an individual's posture. Posture determines whether you lean back or forward, stand straight or hunched. This determines the best line that suits each individual.

L: What do you mean by *line*?

T: It's the hair design that is going to best fit your posture, enhancing or balancing it. Your hair design should balance your posture. You don't want a line that goes forward if a person hunches because it pulls them down even more.

L: Tommy, earlier you mentioned image and the image we should endeavor to create for ourselves. You also mentioned that we are created in God's image, which brings up the fact that you actually have two images. Can you speak to this?

T: I would love to. The two images that everyone has are: (1) the image people see when they look at you, and (2) the image that's inside of you that only God can see. People spend a great deal of time working on their outer image, but they forget their inner image. In fact, the Bible states that "Man looks at the outer appearance, but God looks at the heart" (1 Samuel 16:7). So when we work on our image, it's important to work on both.

L: I agree with you. If we work on our inner image, there is a much more profound impact on our lives, and as the inner beauty grows, our outward appearance is also affected. Improvements made to the inner image are what sustain us and determines true self-worth.

T: Right. As you can see, you must evaluate and assess who you are. What you want to become is up to you. The Bible states that we have been created in God's image. Image originates with Him. What do I mean by this? God is a spirit. We cannot see Him, but each of us is made in His image and have some characteristic of God. There is no one like you. You are unique! You are the best person that can be you!

So why not take a look and evaluate yourself? Look at your greatest assets, and look at your personality. Your personality is who you are. You can enhance that personality, or you can misrepresent yourself by portraying the wrong image.

Your personality has a lot to do with your image. When you're trying to find an image that best suits you, start with your personality as well as your greatest assets. What is your attitude like? Is it negative or positive? Remember, attitude is everything! It determines how you approach creating your image, and your approach determines your results.

Again, you are unique, so develop an image based on that uniqueness, one that will make people look at YOU rather than your imitation of someone else. If you get a new hairstyle or new color, make sure it fits you. Do it for yourself, not someone else. I hope you're getting my point.

L: Tommy, I believe I do. Doing things for oneself takes a paradigm shift in our thinking because so much of our decision-making processes are done based on the way we want others to see us. This has been very enlightening. You've shared things that I've never thought of, and I'm certain this information is going to help a lot of people.

Tommy, let's talk about the shape of an individual's face.

T: This information is so critical because often clients come to the salon with a picture of their favorite celebrity or a photo of a hairstyle, but they don't always see what the trained professional sees. As a professional, I'm checking to see if the style is going to work with their face shape. Just because a style looks good on one doesn't mean it works for all.

Let's say it's a bob style with a part in the center of the head, but our client has a very round face. The client is looking at the overall image. What she sees may fit the individual in the photo, but it may not necessarily fit her. This is because her face shape is round, but the person in the photo may have an oblong face. This hairstyle fits an oblong face, but on the person with the round face, a center part makes the face seem even rounder or larger.

It's critical to consider face shapes because the hairstyle should not accentuate roundness but balance the face shape to give the illusion that it is oval. The whole idea is to give proportion to one's face. A person with a round face is given more balance with an off-center part or with a fringe or bangs with an asymmetrical line. A square bang accentuates the roundness of the face, but an asymmetrical line diminishes the roundness, adding a softer look to the face.

In creating your image, makeup and clothing should also be a consideration, as well as body shape. If a person has a short waist and a round body type, she can create the appearance of a lengthened, narrower waist and broaden her shoulders by carefully choosing her clothes. For instance, wearing a garment with 'v' shaped lines will give the appearance of height.

L: Tommy, this reminds me of line design generally found in fashion.

T: Correct. The whole point is to evaluate the person's features from head to toe in order to enhance assets and minimize what would be considered flaws. Taking into consideration the shape of the nose and size of the lips or ears, among other things, are all practices a trained image maker should look to engage. This is what I do when I'm working with a client or training stylists. The goal is to give the stylist effective techniques and tools that will aide them when they go back to the salon so their clients can look their absolute best.

Unfortunately, many stylists don't consider these factors. They customarily ask the client, "What do you want?" And typically they leave it up to the client rather than educating them. Our goal should be giving professional advice and recommendations based on their facial features and what's really going to accentuate their assets. The reason you go to the professional is for professional advice. Most clients don't actually realize they need assistance in these areas.

I'm not saying we shouldn't listen to the clients or take their opinion seriously. What I am saying is that the professional has been trained and must educate the clients and get them to see what the trained eye sees.

L: So the goal is finding the balance between what the client wants and needs, and the professional's expertise.

T: Exactly. Focusing on client needs is key. I want to get women to appreciate what they have. For example, if your hair is short, don't go out and buy hair to make you happy. Find a trained professional who can take what you have and create a style that enhances your beauty. Make the best of what you have by receiving a great haircut that enhances who you are and accentuates your best assets.

L: Tommy, this concept of face shape is an interesting idea. Can you give a few more examples?

T: Yes. For someone with an oblong-shaped face, which is typically long and narrow, she should select a hairstyle and makeup that complements the face. You can't select hair and makeup that complement a person with an oval face. So in selecting a hairstyle, you have to consider what will make your face appear proportionate. Avoid hairstyles that are high on the top. Hairstyles that are more face-framing are more suitable, as well as a long layered cut with a fringe. This balances the face and doesn't create too much height, making the face appear longer. I hope you can picture what I just described and seek professional advice from someone with expertise who will be able to help capture the beauty of your unique facial structure.

The beauty industry releases new hairstyle, fashion, and makeup trends on a biannual basis. These are great because we are constantly looking for change—however, always consider whether a particular trend suits your facial shape or body type. If it doesn't, you'll need to make adjustments to the looks that will fit your image.

Chapter 5

THE CARE OF
YOUR TEXTURE

In this chapter we begin by talking about the care and maintenance of your hair. In an earlier chapter we touched on the importance of diet, exercise, and adequate amounts of rest to maintain healthy hair, skin, and your physical body. These are all important to help you maintain your hair.

Let's begin with the proper way to cleanse your hair. This may come as a surprise, but you do not wash your hair, you shampoo your hair. It's important to note the difference.

L: I hate it when you spring something new on me. I've never heard that before!

T: There is a difference. When something is washed, it goes through a vigorous and agitated cycle. Clothes are washed, but hair is shampooed. Your hair is delicate, so you want the shampoo to cleanse it, not agitate it. Agitation creates tangles, snarls, and split ends, and it can also affect the cuticle layer of the hair. This concept comes from individuals who feel that if they're not scrubbing their scalp vigorously, they're not really getting the cleansing they need.

The proper way of shampooing the hair is to use the tips of your fingers—not the fingernails—and manipulate the scalp by massaging in order to release any buildup of product or anything on the scalp (dead skin or dandruff). As you massage and manipulate the scalp, the hair should be moved about so that both the hair and the scalp are cleansed. As you shampoo the scalp, you're lifting the hair in your hands to help break down any buildup that may be on the hair. The most important thing is the scalp. A healthy scalp produces healthy hair. And remember, healthy hair is good hair! The lather from the shampoo is what cleanses the hair. It is designed to remove any traces of buildup, so you don't have to be rough when shampooing.

When you're rinsing the hair, you want to make sure you gently lift, separating it to make sure water runs through it. Allow the water to rinse the suds thoroughly rather than using your hands to vigorously agitate it. It's important for us to understand the stress that can often affect the hair. I believe that if hair had nerves, we would feel the pain and sense the stresses we often create for our hair.

I want to touch on the various types of shampoos. There are moisturizing shampoos, protein-based shampoos for body building, shampoos for daily use, and clarifying shampoos. To select the best for your hair type, you must seek a professional to determine which shampoo best meets your needs. We understand this concept in other areas, like seeking out a medical professional to get certain prescriptions for specific ailments. The same holds true for your hair. Just as you wouldn't go into a pharmacy and experiment with various drugs, it is not advisable to purchase just any type of shampoo for your hair. Ask a professional.

Here are just a few things they would consider. Does your hair need moisture? Are you a swimmer? Is your water source hard? Does it come from a well? These are important because if you're a swimmer and have well water or hard water, you would need two types of shampoo: a clarifying (purifying) shampoo to remove chlorine and a moisturizing shampoo to add hydration.

This is important to know because we often choose the wrong shampoo and blame the results on the shampoo, when in reality the product wasn't designed for our particular hair needs. We simply didn't choose the right shampoo.

Here's another key thing to know. You may need to change shampoos based on the season of the year. For example, in the summer when it is extremely humid, you may want to use a protein shampoo that gives your hair body. However, when winter comes and the air is extremely dry, you will need to use a moisturizing shampoo.

I often hear women say, "I've used this shampoo for a long time. Should I switch to another brand?" You don't have to switch to another brand. You may simply need another type of shampoo because the shampoo you're currently using doesn't fit the needs of your hair at that particular time. Your hair needs may fluctuate depending on the condition of the hair, the season of the year, and hormonal changes, etc. You may not need to change brands, just the type of shampoo. Using the proper shampoo for your particular need is critical to the outcome of your hair's condition.

The next step is removing the excess moisture thoroughly from the hair before you apply any type of conditioner. What is a conditioner? A conditioner is product that is used to replace something that the hair is being robbed of or to restore something that the hair needs.

L: Wow! I always thought a conditioner was simply to make my hair soft and easier to comb.

T: It does that too, but it's actually designed to restore what the hair needs.

Let me elaborate. There's so much stress placed on the hair from blow drying, flat irons, chemicals, shampooing, brushing, sun exposure, color treatment, environmental factors, biological factors, medication, worrying, caffeine, and nicotine, just to name a few. Believe it or not, these all put stress on the hair. So do cotton pillowcases, wool hats, and non-silk or non-satin scarves. That's why it's so important to replace what's being robbed from your hair.

Your cuticle layer is the outer layer of the hair, and if viewed under a microscope, it looks like fish scales (healthy cuticle lays flat but damaged cuticle is raised). When that cuticle is damaged, moisture and protein escape, leaving the hair lifeless and dull—not reflecting any shine. That's why it's so important to use conditioners that will restore the hair and mend the cuticle.

The proper way of conditioning the hair is to remove excess moisture by towel drying it, emulsifying (massaging to get the best use of product) the conditioner in your hands, and then blotting it onto the hair. By emulsifying the conditioner, it expands because most professional products are highly concentrated. The result is that you'll actually use less conditioner. Then massage any remaining conditioner on your hand into the hair. For deeper conditioning, you may place a plastic cap over the hair and sit under a dryer for 10-15 minutes. This allows the conditioner to absorb deeper into the hair. You can also follow the manufacturer instructions.

There are different types of conditioners for the hair: (1) protein that gives the hair strength, (2) moisturizing to hydrate the hair, (3) daily use (typically acidifying) to help keep the cuticle intact, and (4) reconstructors that rebuild and restore moisture when the hair is damaged, needing both protein and moisture.

This information on conditioners is so vital because, just like shampoos, knowing the proper type of conditioner to use is critical to the healthiness and condition of your hair.

Some individuals don't know what their hair needs are, so again, it's important to seek the advice of a professional. They are trained in these areas and can give proper guidance based on what the hair needs.

Shampooing and conditioning are only half of what's needed to care for and maintain your hair. Balance comes when we properly care for our total being—spirit, soul, and body. Stresses have to be eliminated, and my personal belief is that it's also important that we learn to pray. Through prayer, God provides peace, comfort, and soundness of mind.

Let's talk about other ways you can take care of your hair, like selecting the correct brush. Inexpensive, plastic brushes tend to scratch, rip, and damage the hair. One of the best types of brushes to use, if you like brushing your hair, is the natural boar-bristle brush. The proper use of the brush, as well as the blow dryer and other styling implements, is essential to caring for your hair.

Proper use of the blower dryer means never using it on hair that is soaking wet. Always remove some of the moisture by towel drying or sitting under a hooded dryer for a few minutes. If you're going to use a hand dryer, always start near your hairline and work your way toward the crown. Never start on top.

L: Why is that?

T: Because when you start on top, you fight through damp hair to dry the hair underneath, damaging it. By starting underneath, drying the hair in smaller sections and bringing down successive sections, it's easier to manage because you're not fighting through wet hair. This method causes less stress on the hair. If you have medium or long hair, you're ripping the hair by starting on top.

When you start from the bottom, you don't have to rip through wet hair. This technique is primarily for medium to long hair. Short hair is a lot easier to blow dry. You have a choice to use your fingers or a brush while blow drying because you have less hair to deal with.

One of the main reasons I mention this technique of drying is because many people use blow dryers due to time constraints. Therefore, it is vital to learn how to properly use your tools to maintain the healthiness of your hair.

Let's talk about different types of products that will help prevent damage to your hair during the styling process. It's very important to use thermal protection. Thermal protectors are products that come in either liquid or oil form, which should be absorbed into the hair. It should not sit on top of the hair. Thermal protectors shield the hair from heat and help to seal the cuticle layer. They also protect the hair whenever you use a blow dryer, flat iron, or any type of heat implement.

L: Can you give me examples of oils considered to be absorbent?

T: Argan oil, olive oil, jojoba oil, and Shea butter, just to name a few.

These are a few of the ingredients found in hair products that manufacturers use in a process that breaks the product into molecule size (making it very tiny) in order to help it absorb into the hair. Olive oil, among others, can be used on the scalp as a hot oil treatment.

After shampooing the hair, apply the oil with a cotton swab directly to the scalp. I recommend using a cotton swab to prevent applying too much oil. After applying the oil, apply your conditioner, cover your head with a plastic cap, and sit under the dryer at medium heat for 10-15 minutes. The oil is for the conditioning of the scalp and the conditioner provides nourishment for the hair. The hot oil treatment can be used for those with dry, flaky scalp. Sitting under heat allows the oil to get into the skin and the conditioner to penetrate deeper into the hair.

When I talk about maintaining the healthiness of hair, I'm speaking about all types and textures of hair. This is critical because regardless of what the texture of your hair is, it's important to know how to maintain it. In an earlier chapter, we talked about *good hair* and *bad hair*. Remember that healthy hair is good hair and damaged hair is bad hair.

Knowing your hair type is going to determine how you should care for your hair. If your hair is straight, your needs will be different from someone with curly hair. However, both types of hair need to be cleansed and conditioned properly, and understanding the types of products that are suitable for your hair texture is the key.

For example, when an individual with curly hair is trying to create a style to make his or her hair straight, more stress is placed on the hair than someone with naturally straight hair. Allow me to elaborate on that statement. Individuals with naturally curly hair who decide they want straight hair have two options: (1) chemical straightening, or

(2) blow drying and flat ironing. This means that the hair is being robbed of vital nutrients and will need to be restored. The hair requires treatments to restore protein, moisture, and essential fatty acids. If these vital nutrients are not restored, the end result will be damaged hair.

If individuals with straight hair decide to curl it, they have three options: (1) perming, (2) roller setting, or (3) curling with a curling iron. Setting the hair is a temporary service that inflicts less stress on the hair. A curling iron will add some stress on the hair, but perming will result in applying the most stress. This is the main reason both types of hair need proper care and replenishing with the vital nutrients that are being removed by chemical and heat processes.

No matter how you are styling your hair, whatever is being removed must be replenished for it to remain healthy.

Imagine someone taking a piece of wood and constantly rubbing it on your hand. Eventually the skin will break, and you will start to bleed and feel intense pain. Your hair doesn't feel pain but definitely shows when it's been worn out. Worn-out hair looks brittle, frizzy, lacks shine, and is rough to the touch with short hairs standing out of place. All of this is the result of too much stress placed on the hair and it being robbed of those nutrients that make it shiny, healthy, and soft. When this type of damage is done to the hair, you don't have to worry about getting a haircut, because eventually you'll get a *free* haircut because it will break off! I use this as an example to get you to visualize what can happen to your hair when you fail to care for it properly.

As you can see, maintaining healthy hair takes time, patience, and a great deal of effort. But do it because you're worth it!

Speaking of healthy hair, I want to reiterate something I shared earlier that I feel is very important. There are many things that negatively affect the condition of the hair. Nicotine, caffeine, and certain types of medication have an effect on your hair. These compounds travel through our bloodstream and eventually into the hair strand, affecting the hair negatively. It is also important to note the fact that hard water deposits have a tendency to be very drying to the hair.

L: Wow! There's so much that we need to learn. I love to swim, but I'm always thinking about my hair. How does chlorine affect the hair?

T: Swimming is a wonderful exercise, but be mindful that chlorine can dry the hair and change its color. Chlorine can give blonde hair a greenish cast. After swimming, use a clarifying (purifying) shampoo to remove the buildup of chlorine from the hair. This type of shampoo is useful for helping remove medication, hard water deposits, mineral deposits, iron, and the like. Be sure to follow up with a moisturizing shampoo and conditioner. Clarifying shampoo is suitable for every hair type.

L: Do all of those elements affect the scalp as well?

T: Yes. A healthy scalp produces healthy hair; therefore, it's important to keep the scalp cleansed and conditioned as well.

L: Explain what you mean by keeping the scalp conditioned.

T: Most people think you only condition the hair, but the scalp needs to be conditioned as well. As I previously stated in our conversation about hot oil treatments, conditioning the scalp means replenishing it with moisture and essential oils.

The scalp must be cleansed properly. The skin on the scalp consists of pores, which are the openings of the skin that the hair grows from. If the pores of the scalp are clogged, certain types of bacteria can develop on the scalp. This leads to damage of the hair follicle, which can result in thinning hair.

L: Yikes! Tommy what causes the pores in the scalp to clog?

T: Pores are clogged by improper cleansing and conditioning.

L: Let's focus more on the scalp. Please elaborate a little bit more on hot oil treatments, more specifically olive oil, because I have heard that some have used olive oils with great results.

T: While there are other types of oil you can use, olive oil is one of the least expensive to condition your scalp. It's great if your budget is tight. Olive oil is light and mimics the natural oils in the hair. It helps replenish and adds softness to the hair. It moisturizes the scalp.

Every person needs essential fatty acids restored, regardless of his or her ethnicity or hair texture, and olive oil will aid in providing what the scalp needs.

L: Tommy, does everyone need a hot oil treatment?

T: Individuals with straight hair who produce natural oils may not need it as much as a person with curly hair. That's why it's so important to receive professional advice to help determine whether you need hot oil treatments.

Depending on your geographical area, especially during winter, moisture evaporates from the body as well as the hair. And if you receive chemical services, such as relaxers, color, or perms, they are drying to the hair and scalp. Your scalp needs to be replenished with essential fatty acids. That's why I'm focusing on the scalp, because the hair grows from the scalp and must be maintained just like the skin. You moisturize your skin, and you should moisturize your scalp.

Generally, individuals will focus on hair but neglect the scalp. It is vitally important to take care of both. We've heard different nationalities say they can shampoo every day and others say they don't. What I want you to think about is this: your hair is like a sponge and it absorbs odors. You would never go a week without washing your face! So when your hair and scalp need to be cleansed, shampoo it. If the shampoo is the proper pH, which is 4.5-5.5, compatible to the acid mantle, then you don't have to be concerned with whether the shampoo is drying to the hair—especially if the shampoo is sulfate-free. The label should indicate *sulfate-free*.

L: What is *sulfate-free?*

T: *Sulfate-free* means there are no harsh detergents stripping or drying the hair. When a shampoo has this label, it can be trusted to be gentle to the hair, and it prevents color from fading.

L: How can a consumer know what a shampoo's pH is?

T: If you purchase your shampoo from a salon, the professional hair designer will be able to tell you the pH balance. If you purchase your shampoo from a department store or other local store, you can do a litmus test to help you determine a shampoo's pH balance. Litmus test papers can be purchased at your local drug store.

I hope you're beginning to realize how important it is to maintain both the hair and scalp. Maintaining the healthiness of your hair and scalp should be one of your top priorities.

You should also be concerned with the products and styling tools you use to finish your hair. Finishing products, styling tools, and techniques can be stressful to the hair if used improperly.

L: Wow, I've learned so much about caring for the hair and scalp. Now let's discuss the difference between short hair and long hair.

T: A person who keeps her hair cut short typically has healthier hair.

L: Why is that?

T: Good question. Individuals with very long hair have had their hair for a long time. For example, if you've been wearing your hair long for a number of years, the hair is considered old. What I mean by *old* is that the hair has aged. There are a few factors that can age the hair: biological (time), chemical, environmental, and thermal. Older hair requires more maintenance to keep it healthy. For those who choose to wear their hair long, it is vitally important for them to have it shaped regularly. I recommend every six to eight weeks. If you wear your hair in a short style, as your new hair is growing in, the old hair is regularly being cut. Hair that is four to six inches away from the scalp is considered aged. The hair closest to the scalp is newest and healthiest. The keratin is stronger and healthier. Regardless of the length of your hair, the key is proper maintenance.

L: What does *shaping the hair* mean?

T: Aha! I knew you would ask that. Shaping the hair is actually cutting the hair. Regardless of whether you take off an eighth-inch or a few inches, the hair should be shaped regularly. Don't be afraid to have it done. Shaping will help eliminate split ends and maintain health, which promotes growth. Split ends lead to breakage, which means you lose length rather than gain length. A shape is a silhouette or a form that gives foundation to a style. No foundation, no style!

We focus so much on having a great look, but we should never forsake healthy hair and a great foundation at the expense of achieving a great style. Both are equally important.

A great haircut complements a person's bone structure, personality, and lifestyle. As a professional, I advocate a great haircut! I'm like one of my teachers, and I quote, "I'm one who cuts the style and not styles the cut." The cut makes the style!

Chapter 6

THE IMAGE IN THE MIRROR

As an image maker, image is one of my favorite topics, because I have the opportunity to help people create their unique persona. Many individuals seek to find their own image, but I believe our image has become distorted because we typically get our ideas of image from the media and try to ascribe those images to ourselves.

I hear this frequently when consulting with clients. They will bring in a photo and say, "This is what I want," or "Oh, I want to look like this celebrity or that one." There is a reason why this happens. People aren't satisfied with themselves. They look at others admiringly and think, "If only I had hair like hers, or were tall like her, or had beautiful eyes and skin like hers." We need to understand what the ideal image is.

One of the greatest books ever written, in my opinion, is the Bible. It tells us all about image. In Genesis 1:26 we learn that God created us in His own image. The Bible also teaches that God is a spirit. With that in mind, although we think we can't physically see the image of God, we actually can simply by looking at mankind. God created us in His image, and what He sees of Himself, He actually gave to us.

Let me elaborate more on this. Customarily, people look on the outer surface rather than looking within. Your true image should start with your character. Once you discover that you are created in God's image, the character of God should reflect the true image of who you really are. Our true image will help us understand what our outer image should be. It is important to learn to appreciate and make the best of what we have been given. Each individual has a uniqueness that no one else possesses. No one can ever be *you* the way you can. You are the best *you* that was ever created.

Let's think about this for a moment. Your features, body structure, and the texture of your hair are unique. What makes your outer image special is what you possess inside. When we look in the mirror and behold our outer appearance, often we're not satisfied with what we see. When we see ourselves in the mirror, we have a tendency to see something that fits another person rather than ourselves. Therefore, our image does not consist of who we really are. It is often a mixture of what we see of others, rather than whom God created us to be and the image we have been given. We need to learn to look at ourselves and appreciate where our true image comes from instead of subscribing to the dictates of society. There are some who have a healthy self-image, but there are many who don't. I've said all this to help you value and embrace what you have been given.

Let's look at skin tone. Your particular skin tone, whether it's light, dark, medium, olive, yellow, brown, or any other color, was given to you for a reason. Skin tone does not make one person more beautiful than another. When we look all around us at nature, we see the many shades of color. My point is that God is a God of creativity. He created the various skin tones to reflect His creativity.

L: I get your point. I remember a time while vacationing in the Bahamas I entered a garden filled with flowers. I exclaimed to my friend, "Wow, God must really love color!" It came out just like that. No forethought and no editing, just appreciation for the beauty that lay before me.

T: That's exactly my point. God created us all with different shades of color to reflect His glory, because everything that was created has color and everything has texture. That brings me to my next point about image, and that is the texture of your hair.

When we look in the mirror at the texture of our hair, we may or may not be pleased with what we see. Some have an image in their mind of what they want to look like, but it is not reality.

Is it wrong to change the texture that we have if we're not happy? I pose this question because some of you will probably think, "Well, if we're to be satisfied and happy with the image that we have, then why do we straighten, perm, or color our hair?" The answer to that is very simple. We change the texture of our hair to have options. You're not changing your image, because remember, your image is within. It's the same with coloring or perming your hair. These are just ways of giving you options. Remember, you don't change your hair because you're trying to duplicate the image of someone else.

For example, coloring your hair will help express your personality, complement your skin tone, and enhance your natural beauty. Changing your hair is an accessory to fashion, at the same time, enhancing the outer image that fits you, not someone else.

The point of all this is to make you aware that often people criticize us when we make changes, but we're doing it to satisfy ourselves and not others. There's nothing wrong with wanting to look your best and enhancing what you have. A perfect example is the refining process of a diamond. A diamond, when first found, does not reflect the natural beauty and value that lies beneath the surface. The natural beauty is uncovered when it is refined. And that's the way it is when we want to enhance our natural beauty. We choose options to reflect the value and beauty that lies within. When we enhance our natural beauty, it reflects our inner creativity.

The next time you look in the mirror, I would like to challenge you to look for the *real* you, not someone else. Concentrate on *your* hair, *your* eyes, *your* nose, *your* lips, *your* cheek bones, and imagine the possibilities. Don't be critical, be creative! Bring out the best you. The only image you should be concerned with is the image you see in the mirror.

Chapter 7

HAIR FASHION

We have to look at hair the way a fashion designer looks at a garment. Every era has its own trends. Remember the bell bottoms of the seventies? The mini skirt, hot pants, and big shoulder pads of the eighties? What types of hairstyles comes to mind? Just as there are fashion trends in clothing, there are also trends in hairstyles.

Remember the shag, the wedge, the savage (sa-vaje)? These hairstyles were popular back in the era when hairstyles had a name, a meaning, and they dictated hair fashion.

L: When did that stop and how?

T: Originally hairstyles were named by famous hair designers to coincide with clothing fashions. Today the trend has shifted from naming individual hairstyles to hair designers developing *collections* of cuts. Every spring and fall new collections are designed to coincide with the latest fashion trends.

Let's think about timeless fashions. Some haircuts stay the same. Just like the little black dress or your favorite cardigan, there are hair fashions that will never go out of style: the classic and graduated bob or the pixie. These are timeless looks that will always be fashionable.

With contemporary hair fashions, we see more texture. We see razor cuts, more asymmetry, choppiness, and disheveled and disconnected looks.

I like to classify hair fashion in five categories: trendy, casual, commercial, classic, and evening. Let me explain the differences.

Trendy styles are typically worn by people who are risk takers. These hairstyles are characteristic of the hip-hop, tattoo, and body piercing cultures, which have their own unique styles. Typically you see more trendy hair fashions in music videos, teen programming, and music award shows. Disheveled, Textured, Asymmetrical, Disconnected

L: Let's go on to casual hair fashion.

T: The casual individuals typically prefer a simple haircut and tend to dress informally. Having a laid-back personality, they want something that requires very little maintenance. This is someone who might prefer a layered cut and styles that are easy to maintain—wash and go. Simple, Clean, Neat

Next is the commercial category. The commercial look refers to someone who is on the cutting edge of fashion. This is someone who wants to make a statement. This look is a cross between classic and trendy. They want something that's fashionable but edgy—a look that can take them from the boardroom to an evening out on the town, something you would see in a magazine that would make you stand out. Edgy, Classic Fused with Trendy

L: Talk about classic. I think I tend to lean toward a classic look.

T: Yes, you do. The classic hair fashion is worn by the woman who is elegant in both her personality and fashion sense. Her hair is typically cut in a precision style where every hair is in place. Precise, Polished, Falls in Place Easily

Now, the evening hair fashion is the upsweep style. These are styles you might see on the *red carpet* that complement expensive gowns and special occasion apparel. Evening hair fashion comprises styles not worn on a daily basis. The French twist or chignons are styles worn with formal or evening wear. You wouldn't wear an after-five evening gown to the office; neither should you wear an evening hairstyle to the office. Formal, Sleek, Elegant

When you analyze these categories, you can see there is a time and place for each one of these styles. So think about the type of clothing fashion an individual would wear and the hair fashion that would complement it. For example, you probably wouldn't see trendy individuals wear an elegant evening style. They'd wear a style that's more risk-taking. Their personality typically dictates the hair fashion they will wear.

To really picture hair fashion, look at some of the trend-setting cities like Chicago, New York, Milan, London, and Paris—all fashion capitals. What do you see? In these cities you will see the creative fusion of clothing and hair, which is the epitome of the fashion world!

When you come into contact with individuals who fit these different categories, you get a sense of their personality and who they are.

L: Is it possible for an individual to have more than one style?

T: Yes, although I believe some may have more than one style because they are trying to be something they're not. In most cases people tend to cater to only one style.

In order to really figure this out, notice the hair fashion in comparison to the clothing style. If they don't complement each other, this individual may need assistance in determining what hairstyle best complements the individual's clothing fashion and vice versa, thus developing their own unique style. For example, if you see someone with a trendy hairstyle wearing conservative or casual clothing, it may be an indication the person isn't sure of what his or her style is.

As we look at hair fashion, think about this: hair fashion and clothing fashion should typically complement each other and also fit the individual's personality. But individuals can move from one category to another, depending on the occasion, without changing who they really are in terms of their personality.

Another important aspect of hair fashion is color, which is indicative of what is appropriate or typical in each hair fashion category. Bold, chunky, bright hair color is typically worn in trendy looks. Hair colors that may clash, like black and platinum or bright red and black don't necessarily complement one another, but when together, they make a statement. Trends contrast.

For the commercial category, you typically see color that is very beautiful—color and highlights together—not chunky and contrasting as in the trendy hair category. Colors that typically complement each other while making a statement are shades of brown, blonde, or copper. Monotones with varying hues are characteristic of this hair fashion category. Caramels, browns, and blondes are often found together. Commercials complement.

The classic category is solid in its color pallet: for example, solid red, copper, brunette, or black. The precision of a bob cut with a solid color is a hallmark of its beauty. Classics conform.

The casual category typically wears very subtle highlights, if any. They don't use a lot of color, and when they do, it tends to be something that's simple and understated. Casuals simplify.

When we think of texture in terms of hair fashion, trendy people wear contrasting textures—hair that's straight in one area and curly in another. Or they'll sport a style that's cut very short in one area and long in another. Trendy individuals typically choose a style with a lot of activity. A great example is a Mohawk, which has a very spiky edge to it.

There is some texture in the commercial category, but not much in the classic category. Texture in this sense refers to the style, not the type of hair. Casuals typically prefer hairstyles that are low maintenance with less activity.

Hair fashion is as important as clothing fashion when it comes to defining and enhancing your image and exuding your personal style.

Chapter 8

MYTH BUSTERS

In this chapter we're going to clear up some of the misconceptions or misunderstandings about hair as well as some of the related stigmas. Some of the questions asked may have been answered in previous chapters, but for the sake of our discussion, I felt it important to address the topic again.

L: I've heard conflicting views on how often a person should shampoo his or her hair. It seems certain races shampoo their hair daily while others can't shampoo their hair more often than once every two weeks. Is that true?

T: This is a myth I would definitely like to address. Individuals should shampoo their hair as often as needed. Let me elaborate. I know it's been said that certain groups of people shampoo their hair often with no problem, and those with excessively curly hair should not shampoo their hair on a weekly basis. Let's start with the European hair. You'll find here in America that Caucasians typically shampoo their hair every day. And the question is, "Why is that?" By removing natural oils and environmental pollutants more often, the hair will have more body, and some people just like that fresh, clean feeling. It's simply a matter of preference.

Typically, people who shampoo their hair on a daily basis produce an abundance of oil from the scalp, and as a result, it leaves the hair flat and unmanageable. If we take a look at women in European countries with the same type of hair, they may go for longer periods of time without shampooing because they like that oily feeling. It's a matter of how they like their hair to perform. Some people like when their hair has some degree of oiliness because they like the way it looks. I'm not saying it's a rule. It truly depends on the individual. Some people like that squeaky clean feeling and some don't. That's what I mean when I say it's a matter of preference. People who shampoo their hair daily say they like its look and manageability. Now, does a person have to shampoo daily? Not necessarily. It's a choice.

The other part of this myth addresses people with excessively curly hair (such as African Americans) who might cleanse their hair weekly or twice monthly. The thought is the hair will become dry or brittle and cause damage if the hair is shampooed often. Additionally, the process of finishing the hair also becomes a challenge for many, thus leading people to buy into the idea of not shampooing regularly.

Believe it or not, there are some with excessively curly hair who shampoo daily or as often as needed. Again, it's not a problem for them to do so. The problem can be in styling the hair. That's where the damage can take place. Depending on the hairstyle, those with excessively curly hair may choose to press, blow dry, flat iron, and/ or use a curling iron for the finished look. The problem is with the heat that accompanies the finishing process. That's where a lot of the dryness and damage takes place. It's not shampooing that causes damage, especially when they use the proper shampoo for their particular hair type.

Years ago, shampoos were formulated with a higher pH, and they were designed to remove oil from the hair. Shampoos were primarily formulated to address the problem of oily hair, so as a result, if it was used by those with excessively curly hair, regardless of race, it dried the hair out. Excessively curly hair has a tendency to be dry. Unlike other types of hair, it lacks natural oil.

The proper pH level of shampoo today is 4.5-5.5 and has been discovered to be compatible to the acid mantle, which are our oil glands. Hair itself does not have a pH level. When the pH level is in that range, it's milder and gentler on the hair. This is where the myth came from that individuals with excessively curly hair shouldn't shampoo their hair daily. It wasn't necessarily the cleansing of the hair but the higher pH level stripping the hair of much needed natural oils.

Those with excessively curly hair may shampoo their hair as often as desired. It depends on how well they can handle their hair after shampooing. The key is to place less stress on their hair. For example, there are techniques one can use to decrease the amount of stress placed on the hair. Those with relaxers may set the hair on rollers or use a technique called wrapping. Using a hooded dryer instead of blow drying is also less stressful on the hair. My point is that it can be done, but the individual must realize you will place more stress on the hair if you don't wear it in its natural state.

L: Tommy, it's my understanding that certain cultures believe the scalp should be oiled. Can you explain that?

T: That is a very good question. Everyone needs oil, regardless of their nationality. Let me explain what I mean by that. Your scalp secretes oil from your sebaceous glands, which are designed to lubricate and protect the hair as well as the scalp. That's why in some cultures you find that women shampoo their hair daily, especially here in America. In this country, you have a diverse group of people. The majority of Caucasians shampoo their hair daily because typically their oil glands produce more oil because of how the hair strand grows out of the scalp. Let me emphasize what I mean. Let's take excessively curly hair as an example. Typically this type of hair is found among African Americans. Now there's a vast difference between how straight hair and excessively curly hair grows out of the scalp.

Hair that's straight grows out of the scalp more rounded, and, therefore, the oils can travel up from the scalp more easily than hair that's very, very curly, which grows out flat. Hair that grows out flat prevents the oil from reaching the ends because of the angle at which it emerges from the scalp. Within this hair type, the scalp does not have as many oil glands, therefore, this type of hair and scalp are not easily naturally lubricated because of the lack of oil. Moreover, the hair has the tendency to be drier.

People may use oils to help compensate for the lack of natural oils; however, the oils that should be used are those that are absorbed and useful for lubrication, not heavy greases as they cause the hair to become dirty. Everyone needs some form of oil in the hair. It serves as protection and lubrication for the hair and scalp. Some types of chemical services and shampoos are harsh and deplete the hair of essential fatty acids, without which the hair is dry and lacks shine.

The problem is that the products we use on our hair strip the hair of oils. Heavy greases sit on top of the hair and collect debris, causing the hair to become dirty. Hot oil treatments are designed to condition the scalp. They serve a greater purpose as opposed to someone taking heavy greases and applying them directly to the scalp. You can use light oil that absorbs into the hair and scalp, but the best method of scalp lubrication would be a hot oil treatment. The molecules must be small enough to absorb into the hair and scalp. If they are too large, they sit on the surface of the scalp, causing buildup and a flattened hairstyle. Hopefully, this will end the myth of greasing the scalp.

L: Here's another myth. Have you ever heard that when a woman is pregnant, she's not supposed to shampoo her hair?

T: This is definitely a myth. It's an old wives tale that's been passed from generation to generation. There is no scientific proof that a pregnant woman cannot shampoo her hair. People felt that if you shampooed your hair while pregnant, you'd catch a cold because your pores were open. It's just an old wives' tale that's been propagated. I've shampooed many pregnant women's hair and they didn't *catch a cold*. Colds are caused by a virus.

L: What about the myth that a *little dirt* actually helps the hair grow?

T: No, a little dirt does not help the hair grow. You want your scalp to be clean because a healthy scalp produces healthy hair. More importantly, your scalp is part of your face, and you wouldn't go weeks without washing your face.

L: I've never thought of my scalp as part of my face.

T: Yes, it is. Did you know that an unclean scalp and hair can aggravate acne and cause skin problems? Think about it. If your hair is heavily soiled, and you lie on your pillow every night, that soiled pillowcase is coming into direct contact with your facial skin.

L: Wow! You're right. So you're just basically lying in a pile of dirt!

T: Well, I don't know if I'd quite put it that way. I'll tell you something else I've noticed in the salon. People who wear bangs and aren't shampooing enough usually have some type of skin problem on their forehead. So again, people should shampoo their hair as often as necessary, or at least weekly, and use the proper shampoo for their hair type.

Think about it this way, your hair is like a sponge and absorbs whatever is in the surrounding environment. For instance, if you're cooking or in a smoked-filled room, your hair will absorb those odors.

In my line of work, when I apply chemical services to an individual's hair, the cuticle layer opens and exposes the odors in the hair, such as fish, pancakes, grilling, cigarette smoke, bacon, etc. These odors are exposed because they are trapped in unclean hair. Suppose you took a shower and didn't wash certain parts. Although you took a shower, you're not really clean, and you are going to have bad body odor. Your scalp produces odors too. When a person hugs you, you want them to know you have proper hygiene. As you see, it's so important that we properly cleanse our hair on a regular basis.

L: Tommy, I've always heard that when a woman is pregnant, her hair grows more than usual. Is this true? And if so, why is that?

T: That's a very good question because over the years I have come into contact with so many women who were expecting and they experience so many different changes. It's very interesting that most doctors won't explain or let their patients know what's going to happen with their hair during this time period.

L: That is interesting because the doctor tells you just about everything that's going to happen with your body, but the subject of hair never comes up. I bet a lot of them don't even think about it.

T: It's extremely important to women because they are very sensitive about their hair during this time. A large percentage of pregnant women experience faster hair growth, their skin has a glow, and their nails are stronger. This is all by design because their estrogen level increases, and in most cases, they are taking prenatal vitamins, which also contributes to increased hair growth.

After the birth, when the baby is between three and five months old, the mother may experience further changes with her hair. This change is *not* so good. The hair starts to thin out in the temple area and sheds more, and this is usually when she starts to panic.

L: Why is this happening?

T: The estrogen level is starting to return to normal and the hormones are beginning to adjust. This experience usually lasts about a month and depends on how well the individual maintains her diet and vitamin intake. I've seen women who experience significant hair loss and some minimal loss. A vast majority of my post partum clients do experience some type of hair loss. And my advice to them is, "Don't panic! You won't go bald." It's just something that naturally takes place. During the time when the estrogen level was elevated, the hair didn't shed a lot. It was very healthy. Following birth, increased shedding occurs as estrogen returns to normal. The shedding will level out.

L: Here's another myth. I heard you're not supposed to shampoo your hair for two weeks after a chemical service. Is that true?

T: Actually, it's false. It's been stated that if individuals receive perm services, they're not supposed to shampoo for three days. If the perm was successfully done, you can shampoo right away. However, you always want to use a low pH level shampoo, between 4.5 and 5.5, that is sulfate-free. Most individuals were afraid that the curl may slightly relax after shampooing, but that's not true. You can successfully shampoo right away if you use a shampoo specially formulated for chemically-treated hair with a low pH level.

As far as relaxers are concerned, there's no truth that one must wait to shampoo. Whether the relaxer straightened successfully or not, the most important factor is that the entire caustic residue be thoroughly removed from the hair.

In terms of hair color, redheads have a tendency to fade quicker than all of the other shades. To prolong the color with all hair color, it's important to use a sulfate-free shampoo; then you don't have to worry about any color being stripped from the hair. Sulfate-free shampoos are gentler on the hair, and they are color safe. You can find sulfate-free shampoo in most salons. So you can shampoo after a chemical service, but be aware of the type of shampoo you use.

L: When should you cut a baby's hair? I heard that cutting a baby's hair causes the texture to change.

T: This is a subject that may be sensitive to some ethnic groups. I've heard in some ethnicities that a child's hair should not be cut until after one or two years of age because you may affect the texture of the child's hair.

In actuality, you cannot affect something that has already been genetically determined. Children receive hair texture based on the genetics of their parents. Whatever the texture is going to be, it already is. For example, you may have one parent with curly hair and the other with straight hair. Their child may have a combination of both of those textures. Or you may have parents who both have straight hair, so the chances of that child having very curly hair are slim. But there are some cases where the ancestors may have a hair texture that is different from their offspring and skips a generation, possibly manifesting in their grandchild. So to really answer your question, no one needs to worry about cutting their child's hair before age one or at any other time. Whatever the texture of the child's hair will be is genetically predisposed.

Some children are born with a lot of hair, some with very little, and some with fine hair, but over time, the texture will change in accordance with that child's genetic predisposition. Children are born with immature hair. Over time it will fall out, and the true texture of the hair will grow in.

L: I've heard that wearing the hair braided causes it to grow. Is that true?

T: This is a very sensitive topic because so many people think braids are the answer to their hair dilemmas. Braiding in and of itself is not bad. It does, however, depend on how it is done. Let me be very specific on how I address this issue. When the braids are braided loose and larger, there is less stress on the scalp and hair. Where I would caution a person is in braiding chemically relaxed hair. When you braid hair that's chemically relaxed, taking very thin sections and braiding it tightly, you are doing extreme damage to the hair. And the reason is that relaxed hair is already in a weakened state, and when you braid it extremely tightly, you're placing a lot of stress and tension on the hair, and its integrity is jeopardized. This will cause hair breakage and hair loss.

Let me give you an analogy that I used in an earlier chapter that I think is quite fitting for this subject. Hair is very much like fabric. Fabric can be worn and ripped and become very frail if not handled properly. Denim is very strong, but if a child is constantly crawling on his knees, he will wear the denim out, and you'll notice the shredding and ripping in the knees. This is very similar to what happens to chemically treated hair when it's braided extremely tightly and worn in that style over a period of time.

When the hair is braided so tightly that the skin is pulled taut, you will negatively affect the hair and damage the follicle, which may result in alopecia or baldness. Once the hair follicle is damaged, permanent hair loss will occur. So to answer the question of whether braiding makes the hair grow—no, the braiding doesn't make the hair grow. The reason some people will notice growth after their hair has been braided is because the hair was in somewhat of a resting stage, but the tightly-braided hair is being stressed and tortured, and you won't see the results until the braids are removed. That's when you will notice the thinness of the hair. Even though you may have some growth, you'll still have thinness, damage, and breakage of the hair. It defeats the purpose.

L: I've heard that pulling the hair back in a ponytail is bad for the hair. I've always just thought of it as quick, easy styling.

T: There is some truth to it being an easy style. However, you will see some thinning and breakage at the hairline over a period of time because of constantly pulling the hair back. You're placing a lot of stress on the hair, and the hair around the hairline is much more fragile. Research shows the medulla, one of the layers of the hair shaft, is missing around the hairline. This is why some women experience balding around the hairline. You have to be very careful with the amount of stress you apply to the hair.

L: Is this applicable for all hair types?

T: Yes.

L: I've always heard the best way to choose hair dressers is by the way they style hair. Is that valid?

T: There is more tha n one component you should consider when choosing a professional hair dresser. Yes, you do want someone who's creative, skillful, and knowledgeable in terms of cutting, coloring, perming, and relaxing. But the most important attribute of a hair professional is that person's knowledge of hair. Do they *really* know hair? And when I say hair, I'm talking about *all* textures and how to properly care for it.

Consider how well they evaluate the specific dynamics of your hair and communicate your hair care needs. Are they equally concerned with the condition of your hair as well as the style? This is why it's so important for the professional to give the client a consultation prior to working with the hair. They need to know the client's hair history. They need to know what chemicals have been used on the client's hair in past. Do they take medications? What is their current lifestyle? This information is needed prior to a professional working with your hair, and a good, licensed professional will take these measures to ensure that your hair is properly cared for.

Most people think if the hair dresser is very creative, if they can really style hair and make it look good, that these qualities epitomize a great hair dresser. They forget about the other components that define a true professional. It's a combination of everything I mentioned. The hair professional must be able to meet the needs of the client. He or she is there to serve the client regardless of what the needs are.